OSTEOPENIA

A Beginner's Quick Start Guide for
Women on Managing Osteopenia Through
Diet and Other Natural Methods, With
Sample Recipes and a Meal Plan

Mary Golanna

mindplusfood

CONTENTS

Title Page

Copyright

Introduction   4

Chapter 1: All About Osteopenia   5

Chapter 2: Osteopenia and Osteoporosis   11

Chapter 3: Managing Osteopenia Through Natural Means   14

Chapter 4: Osteopenia and Diet   19

Conclusion   41

Disclaimer

By reading this disclaimer, you are accepting the terms of the disclaimer in full. If you disagree with this disclaimer, please do not read the guide.

All of the content within this guide is provided for informational and educational purposes only, and should not be accepted as independent medical or other professional advice. The author is not a doctor, physician, nurse, mental health provider, or registered nutritionist/dietician. Therefore, using and reading this guide does not establish any form of a physician-patient relationship.

Always consult with a physician or another qualified health provider with any issues or questions you might have regarding any sort of medical condition. Do not ever disregard any qualified professional medical advice or delay seeking that advice because of anything you have read in this guide. The information in this guide is not intended to be any sort of medical advice and should not be used in lieu of any medical advice by a licensed and qualified medical professional.

The information in this guide has been compiled from a variety of known sources. However, the author cannot attest to or guarantee the accuracy of each source and thus should not be held liable for any errors or omissions.

You acknowledge that the publisher of this guide will not be held liable for any loss or damage of any kind incurred as a result of this guide or the reliance on any information provided within this guide. You acknowledge and agree that you assume all risk and responsibility for any action you undertake in response to the information in this guide.

Using this guide does not guarantee any particular result (e.g., weight loss or a cure). By reading this guide, you acknowledge that there are no guarantees to any specific outcome or results you can expect.

All product names, diet plans, or names used in this guide are for identification purposes only and are the property of their respective owners. The use of these names does not imply endorsement. All other trademarks cited herein are the property of their respective owners.

Where applicable, this guide is not intended to be a substitute for the original work of this diet plan and is, at most, a supplement to the original work for this diet plan and never a direct substitute. This guide is a personal expression of the facts of that diet plan.

Where applicable, persons shown in the cover images are stock photography models and the publisher has obtained the rights to use the images through license agreements with third-party stock image companies.

INTRODUCTION

If you have osteopenia, it means that your bone density is lower than normal. Osteopenia is not as severe as osteoporosis, but it does increase your risk of developing osteoporosis.

Osteopenia is often diagnosed when a bone density test shows that your bone mineral density (BMD) is lower than it should be. BMD is a measure of how much calcium and other minerals are in your bones.

Osteopenia can occur at any age, but it is most common in older adults. Women are more likely to develop osteopenia than men.

If you have osteopenia, your bone density is lower than normal but not low enough to be classified as osteoporosis. Osteopenia does not cause any symptoms, but it does increase your risk of developing osteoporosis.

In this beginner's quick start guide, you will discover…
- The basics of osteopenia
- The difference between osteoporosis and osteopenia
- How to manage osteopenia through natural methods
- How to manage osteopenia through diet
- Sample recipes

CHAPTER 1: ALL ABOUT OSTEOPENIA

Osteopenia is a condition characterized by loss of bone mineral density (BMD). A lower BMD means that your bones have lost minerals, such as calcium.

When you have osteopenia, your bones are not as strong as they should be. This puts you at risk for fractures.

The bones in your body are made up of many different minerals, including calcium, phosphorus, and magnesium.

These minerals are important for keeping your bones strong and healthy. Calcium is the most abundant mineral in your bones, and it helps to keep them hard and strong. Phosphorus helps to make your bones dense and strong, and magnesium helps to keep your bones healthy and flexible.

Calcium is a mineral that is necessary for many functions in the body, including building and maintaining bones. Bones are constantly being remodeled, with old bone being removed and new bone being formed. Calcium is essential for this process to occur properly.

If you don't get enough calcium in your diet, your body will take calcium from your bones to ensure that your blood levels of calcium remain constant. This can lead to weak and brittle bones, a condition known as osteoporosis.

Phosphorus is essential for building and maintaining strong

bones. It works closely with calcium to promote bone growth and mineralization. Without adequate phosphorus, bones can become weak and brittle. A diet rich in phosphorus is important for people of all ages, but it's especially critical for growing children and teens. Older adults also need to make sure they're getting enough phosphorus to help prevent osteoporosis.

Magnesium is one of the many minerals that your body needs to function properly. It plays a role in over 300 different biochemical reactions in your body, including helping to maintain normal muscle and nerve function, keeping your heart rhythm steady, and supporting a healthy immune system. Magnesium is also important for maintaining proper blood sugar levels and blood pressure.

One of magnesium's most important functions is helping to keep your bones healthy and strong. Magnesium helps to regulate calcium metabolism and is necessary for the formation of bone. It also helps to keep bones flexible by maintaining their collagen content. Magnesium deficiency has been linked with an increased risk of osteoporosis, so getting enough magnesium is essential for bone health.

Symptoms
Osteopenia does not cause any symptoms until a bone fracture occurs or until it reaches Osteoporosis. At that point, you may experience pain and swelling at the site of the fracture.

If a bone breaks (fractures), it can take weeks or months to heal properly. If the bone doesn't heal properly, you may be at risk for further fractures. The best way to determine if you have osteopenia or osteoporosis is to get a bone density test.

Causes of Osteopenia
The most common cause of osteopenia is aging. As you get older, your bones gradually lose minerals, making them weaker. This process is called bone loss. Normally, even in healthy individuals, it's not atypical for bone density to decrease each year.

There are many reasons why bone loss can occur faster than normal:

- A lack of calcium or vitamin D

Calcium is a mineral that is found naturally in food. It is essential for maintaining strong bones and teeth. Calcium is also needed for proper muscle contraction, nerve function, and blood clotting.

Most of the calcium in our bodies is stored in our bones and teeth. When we don't get enough calcium from our diet, our bodies take calcium from our bones, which can lead to weak, brittle bones. This can increase the risk of fractures, particularly in older adults.

Getting enough calcium is important for everyone, but it's especially important for people who are at risk of osteoporosis, a condition that causes bones to become weak and break easily.

Vitamin D is a nutrient that helps the body absorb calcium and phosphate from the diet, which is needed for healthy bones. Vitamin D deficiency can lead to bone problems such as rickets in children, and osteomalacia in adults.

- Smoking

Smoking can lead to bone loss because it impairs the ability of bones to repair themselves.

Smoking also increases the risk of developing osteoporosis, a condition in which bones become fragile and more likely to break.

If you smoke, quitting will improve your bone health. Quitting smoking is one of the best things you can do for your health.

Smoking breaks down bones by affecting the body's ability to absorb calcium. Calcium is essential for healthy bones, and smoking interferes with the body's ability to absorb this important mineral.

In addition, smoking also increases the amount of calcium that is excreted through urine. Over time, this can lead to bone loss and an increased risk of fractures.

- Excessive alcohol and caffeine consumption

There are a few potential mechanisms by which alcohol and caffeine could lead to bone loss. First, both substances can lead to dehydration, and dehydration has been linked with reduced bone density.

Alcohol and caffeine can also both interfere with the body's absorption of calcium, which is essential for healthy bones. Additionally, chronic use of either substance can lead to an increased risk of falls, which can lead to fractures.

While moderate consumption of alcohol and caffeine is not likely to cause bone loss, it's best to limit your intake to avoid any potential negative effects on your health.

- Sedentary lifestyle

A sedentary lifestyle can lead to bone loss because it results in reduced muscle mass and strength. Strong muscles help to protect bones and prevent fractures. Additionally, a sedentary lifestyle can lead to weight gain, which can also contribute to bone loss.

Being overweight or obese puts you at risk for developing osteoarthritis, a condition in which the cartilage that cushions your joints breaks down. This can lead to pain, stiffness, and swelling in the joints.

- Certain medications, such as prednisone

Prednisone is a man-made corticosteroid medication that is used to treat a variety of conditions including allergies, skin conditions, ulcerative colitis, arthritis, lupus, psoriasis, and breathing disorders.

A corticosteroid is a type of steroid that is produced naturally by the body. Corticosteroids are involved in a wide range of activities in the body, including the stress response, immune system function, and inflammation.

Steroids are a class of organic compounds that includes natural and synthetic hormones. Anabolic steroids, which are also known as anabolic-androgenic steroids (AAS), are a type of steroid that helps to promote muscle growth and development.

Corticosteroids can also be made synthetically in laboratories. Synthetic corticosteroids are similar to corticosteroids produced naturally by the body, but they are typically more potent. Corticosteroids are used medically to treat a variety of conditions, including allergies, asthma, autoimmune disorders, and skin conditions.

Corticosteroids are available in a variety of formulations, including creams, ointments, tablets, and injections. Corticosteroids can be taken orally, applied to the skin, or injected into a joint or muscle.

Prednisone can be taken orally as a pill or tablet, or it can be injected into a muscle. Common side effects of prednisone include headache, dizziness, sleep problems, stomach upset, and increased appetite.

There are a few different reasons why prednisone may lead to bone loss. One reason is that prednisone can interfere with the body's ability to absorb calcium.

Prednisone may also increase the breakdown of bone tissue. Additionally, prednisone can reduce the levels of vitamin D in the body, which is important for maintaining healthy bones.

Finally, long-term use of prednisone can suppress the production of hormones that are necessary for bone growth and maintenance. All of these factors can contribute to the development of osteoporosis.

Diagnosis
Osteopenia is often diagnosed when a bone density test shows that your BMD is lower than it should be. BMD is a measure of how

much calcium and other minerals are in your bones. Bones are composed of minerals, water, and collagen. The most abundant mineral in your bones is calcium.

When you have osteopenia, it means that your bones have lost minerals, typically calcium. This can make your bones weaker and more likely to break.

Osteopenia is diagnosed using a bone density test. A bone density test is a type of X-ray that measures how much calcium and other minerals are in your bones.

The most common type of bone density test is dual-energy X-ray absorptiometry (DEXA). DEXA scans are quick and painless. They are usually done on the lower spine and hip because these bones are most likely to break in people with osteoporosis.

During a DEXA scan, you will lie on your back on an X-ray table. A special X-ray machine will pass over your body and take pictures of your bones. The pictures will be used to measure the density of your bones.

If your bone density test shows that you have osteopenia, it does not necessarily mean that you will develop osteoporosis. However, it does mean that you are at an increased risk of developing the condition.

Studies have shown that women over 65 years of age are recommended to take a bone density test.

CHAPTER 2: OSTEOPENIA AND OSTEOPOROSIS

Osteopenia is different from osteoporosis. Osteoporosis is a more serious condition that causes your bones to weaken to the point where they can break easily.

This can lead to an increased risk of fractures, especially in the hip, spine, and wrist. Osteopenia is less serious than osteoporosis, but it can still lead to an increased risk of fractures. Additionally, not everyone with osteopenia will develop osteoporosis.

Women and Osteopenia
While Osteopenia can affect both men and women, it is more common in women. For example, of the 10 million Americans that have Osteoporosis, around 80 percent are women. There are several reasons for this.

First, women tend to have smaller and thinner bones than men. One possible reason for this is that women generally have lower levels of testosterone, a hormone that helps to maintain bone mass. Testosterone helps to maintain bone density by stimulating the production of new bone cells.

It also helps to reduce the rate at which existing bone cells are broken down. This means that testosterone can help to prevent conditions such as osteoporosis, which is characterized by thinning and weakening of the bones.

Additionally, hormones play a role in bone growth. Estrogen, a hormone that decreases during menopause, helps to maintain bone density. Estrogen is a hormone that plays an important role in the development and function of the female reproductive system. Estrogen levels fluctuate throughout a woman's menstrual cycle, and can also be affected by a pregnancy, menopause, and certain medications. Too much or too little estrogen can cause problems with menstruation, fertility, and other aspects

Estrogen plays an important role in bone health. It helps to regulate calcium metabolism and to maintain bone density. Estrogen also affects the cardiovascular system. It helps to regulate blood pressure and to keep the lining of the blood vessels healthy.

When estrogen levels decrease during menopause, the risk of developing osteoporosis increases. This is because, without estrogen to help regulate calcium metabolism, bone loss can occur. Additionally, decreased estrogen levels can lead to an increased risk of cardiovascular disease.

To reduce your risk of developing osteopenia or osteoporosis, it is important to get enough calcium and vitamin D. Calcium is the main mineral that makes up bone. Vitamin D helps your body absorb calcium.

You can get calcium from dairy products, leafy green vegetables, and certain types of fish. You can also take calcium supplements. Vitamin D is found in fortified milk, fatty fish, and exposure to sunlight. You can also take vitamin D supplements.

If you are a woman over the age of 50, it is important to get a bone density test to check for osteopenia or osteoporosis.

In the next few chapters, we will discuss certain foods that can help add more calcium to your diet as well as the different types of exercise that can help to strengthen your bones.

CHAPTER 3: MANAGING OSTEOPENIA THROUGH NATURAL MEANS

There are several lifestyle changes you can make to help prevent the progression of osteopenia to osteoporosis.

One of these ways is through weight-bearing and resistance exercises.

These types of exercises help to build and maintain muscle mass and bone density.

Examples of weight-bearing exercises include walking, running, stair climbing, tennis, and dancing. Resistance exercises help to build muscle mass and can be done with free weights, weight machines, or resistance bands.

It is important to consult with your doctor before starting any new exercise program. This is especially important if you have any existing health conditions or injuries.

If you're starting a walking program from scratch, aim to walk for at least 30 minutes on most days of the week. You can break up your time into shorter stints if that's easier for you, and gradually work up to longer walks as you become more fit.

If you have any health concerns, check with your doctor before beginning a walking program. And be sure to warm up with some easy walking before starting your walk at a moderate or brisk pace.

Here are a few other tips for getting the most out of your walking workouts:

- Wear comfortable shoes that fit well and provide good support.
- Walk with good posture, keeping your head up and shoulders relaxed.
- Swing your arms as you walk to help pump up your heart rate.
- Focus on taking steps with your heel striking the ground first, rolling through to your toe.
- If you're walking outdoors, beware of uneven surfaces, potholes, and other obstacles. Also, be aware of traffic if you're walking on busy streets.
- To help stay motivated, listen to music or audiobooks while you walk, or find a walking buddy.

In addition to exercise, there are several other lifestyle changes you can make to help prevent the progression of osteopenia. These include:

Quitting smoking
Quitting smoking is one of the best things you can do for your health. There are many ways to quit, and no single method is right for everyone. Talk with your doctor about which quitting method might be right for you.

Besides helping to prevent the onset of osteoporosis, there are many other benefits:

- Improved lung health
- Reduced risk of cancer
- Reduced risk of heart disease

- Saving money

If you're ready to quit smoking, there are a few things you can do to increase your chances of success:

1. Choose a date to quit and stick to it. Remove all cigarettes and ashtrays from your home, car, and workplace. Tell your family, friends, and co-workers that you're quitting.

2. Develop a plan to deal with cravings and tough situations. Avoid places where you used to smoke, and have a list of activities to do when you get the urge to smoke.

3. Talk to your doctor about medications that can help you quit smoking. There are many safe and effective options available.

4. Get support from family, friends, or a support group. Quitting smoking is easier with the help of others.

5. Be prepared for setbacks. Don't be discouraged if you have a slip-up—just get back on track and continue working towards your goal of quitting smoking for good!

Reducing your risk of falling by making your home safe and removing any potential hazards

Most people are aware of the obvious dangers in their homes, such as exposed electrical outlets, loose stairs, and cluttered floors. However, many potential hazards are often overlooked. By taking the time to identify and remove these hazards, you can make your home much safer for everyone.

1. Check for loose railings and handrails. These are a common hazard, especially on stairs. Make sure all railings are securely attached to the wall or floor and that there are no loose screws or bolts.

2. Inspect any window coverings in your home. Curtains and blinds can pose a serious strangulation risk, so make sure they are hung properly and free of any loose cords.

3. Be sure to secure any large pieces of furniture to the wall. Dressers, bookshelves, and armoires can tip over easily, especially if they are not properly secured. To prevent this from happening, use brackets or straps to secure these pieces of furniture to the wall.

4. Inspect all of the electrical outlets in your home. Exposed outlets are a serious shock hazard, so make sure they are properly covered. If you have any loose or exposed wires, be sure to have an electrician take a look at them as soon as possible.

5. Keep clutter off the floors and stairs. Clutter can be a trip hazard, so be sure to store items in a safe place. If you have small children, be sure to keep any potentially dangerous items (such as cleaning supplies) out of their reach.

By taking the time to identify and remove potential hazards in your home, you can make it a much safer place for everyone.

Limiting alcohol intake
If you're struggling with limiting alcohol or even struggle with some degree of alcoholism, quitting drinking may seem like an impossible feat. But it's important to remember that recovery is always possible. There are a variety of effective treatment options and support groups available to help you on your journey to sobriety.

Here are a few tips to help you stop drinking:
1. Set realistic goals. If you're not ready to quit completely, set a goal to reduce your alcohol intake. Gradually cutting back will help you reduce your dependence on alcohol and make it easier to eventually stop drinking altogether.

2. Avoid triggers. Make a list of the people, places, and things that trigger your urge to drink. Then, do your best to avoid these triggers. This may mean avoiding social situations where you know alcohol will be present or staying away from bars and clubs.

3. Keep track of your progress. Each day that you don't drink, make a note of it in a journal or calendar. Seeing the days add up can help give you a sense of accomplishment and keep you motivated to stay on track.

4. Seek professional help. If you're struggling to quit drinking on your own, consider seeking professional help. A therapist or counselor can provide you with support and guidance as you work to overcome your addiction.

5. Join a support group. There are many Alcoholics Anonymous (AA) and other support groups available to help people struggling with alcoholism. Attending meetings can provide you with invaluable support and motivation as you work to quit drinking.

These lifestyle changes can help to prevent the progression of osteopenia to osteoporosis. Making these changes early on can help to reduce your risk of developing osteoporosis later in life.

CHAPTER 4: OSTEOPENIA AND DIET

Generally, the following are some high-level principles to follow in terms of eating for osteopenia management:

1. Eat a well-balanced diet that includes a variety of nutrients.

2. Make sure you're getting enough calcium and vitamin D. These two nutrients are essential for bone health. Good sources of calcium include dairy products, leafy green vegetables, and canned fish with bones (such as sardines and salmon). Vitamin D can be found in fatty fish, eggs, and fortified milk.

3. Eat foods rich in vitamin K. Vitamin K helps your body use calcium to build strong bones. Good sources of vitamin K include dark leafy greens, broccoli, and cabbage.

4. Limit salt intake. Too much salt can cause calcium to be excreted from the body, which can lead to osteoporosis. Try to limit your salt intake to 2,000 milligrams per day or less.

Foods to Avoid
- Processed foods, such as lunch meats, hot dogs, and bacon
- Sugar-sweetened beverages, such as soda and energy drinks
- Refined carbohydrates, such as white bread and pasta
- Alcohol
- Caffeine

- Salty Foods
- Spinach may have oxalates, which can reduce calcium absorption.
- Beans may have phytates, which can bind to calcium and reduce absorption.

Foods to Eat

List of Foods with Calcium
- Milk
- Cheese
- Yogurt
- Canned fish with bones (sardines, salmon)
- Dark leafy greens (kale, collards)
- Broccoli
- Cabbage

List of Foods with Vitamin D
- Egg yolks
- Fortified milk
- Fortified cereals
- Fortified orange juice
- Fatty fish (salmon, tuna, mackerel)
- Mushrooms
- List of foods with Vitamin K
- Dark leafy greens (kale, collards)
- Broccoli
- Cabbage

List of Foods with Vitamin K
- Kale
- Brussel sprouts
- Collard greens

A 3-Week Plan

Here is a sample 3 -week plan to help you get started on managing your osteopenia through diet:

Week 1	1. Cut out processed foods, sugary drinks, and refined carbs.
	2. Eat at least 2 servings of calcium-rich foods each day.
	3. Eat at least 2 servings of vitamin D-rich foods each day.
	4. Eat at least 2 servings of vitamin K-rich foods each day.
	5. Limit your salt intake to 2,000 milligrams per day or less.
Week 2	1. Continue to avoid processed foods, sugary drinks, and refined carbs.
	2. Eat 3-4 servings of calcium-rich foods each day.
	3. Eat 3-4 servings of vitamin D-rich foods each day.
	4. Eat 3-4 servings of vitamin K-rich foods each day.
	5. Limit your salt intake to 1,500 milligrams per day or less.
Week 3	1. Continue to avoid processed foods, sugary drinks, and refined carbs.
	2. Eat 4-5 servings of calcium-rich foods each day.
	3. Eat 4-5 servings of vitamin D-rich foods each

day.

	4. Eat 4-5 servings of vitamin K-rich foods each day.
	5. Limit your salt intake to 1,000 milligrams per day or less.

7-Day Meal Plan

Here is a meal plan you can either follow or modify according to your preference.

	Morning	Lunch	Dinner
Day 1	Greek Yogurt Parfait with Berries and Almonds	Salmon with Avocados and Brussels Sprout	Healthy Broccoli with Cheese Sauce
Day 2	Banana Ginger Smoothie	Cauliflower Rice with Chicken and Broccoli	Roasted Mushroom Soup
Day 3	Avocado and Egg Salad	Broccoli-Kale with Avocado Toppings Rice Bowl	Exotic Empanadas
Day 4	Greek Yogurt Parfait with Berries and Almonds	Spicy Tuna Salad	Salmon with Sweet Potato and Kale
Day 5	Pomegranate Refreshing Smoothie	No-Fuss Tuna Casserole	Broccoli Soup
Day 6	Healthy Broccoli with Cheese Sauce	Exotic Empanadas	Salmon with Avocados and Brussels Sprout
Day 7	Fried Eggs and Vegetables	Stir-Fried Cabbage and Apples	Broccoli-Kale with Avocado Toppings Rice Bowl

Sample Recipes

<u>Calcium-Rich Recipes</u>

Greek Yogurt Parfait with Berries and Almonds

Ingredients:
- 1 cup Greek yogurt
- 1 cup mixed berries
- 1/4 cup almonds, chopped
- 2 tbsp. honey

Instructions:
1. In a bowl, combine Greek yogurt, berries, almonds, and honey.
2. Enjoy as is or refrigerate for later.

This recipe features Greek yogurt, which is rich in calcium and protein. The berries provide vitamin C while the almonds provide vitamin E and magnesium.

Cauliflower Rice with Chicken and Broccoli

Ingredients:
- 1 broccoli head
- 1 cauliflower head
- 2 chicken breasts, boneless and skinless
- 1 tbsp. olive oil
- salt
- pepper

Instructions:
1. Preheat the oven to 350°F.
2. Cut the broccoli into small florets.
3. Remove the core from the cauliflower and chop it into small pieces.
4. In a food processor, pulse the cauliflower until it resembles rice.
5. In a baking dish, combine the broccoli, cauliflower rice, chicken, and olive oil. Season with salt and pepper.
6. Bake for 20-25 minutes, or until the chicken is cooked through.

This recipe features chicken, broccoli, and cauliflower rice, all of which are good sources of protein. The broccoli provides calcium and vitamin K while the cauliflower rice is a low-carbohydrate alternative to traditional rice.

Banana Ginger Smoothie

Ingredients:
- 2 pcs. ripe bananas
- 2 cups milk
- 1 cup yogurt
- 1/2 cup ice
- 1/2 tsp. garlic, peeled and shredded
- Optional: 2 tbsp. honey or brown sugar

Instructions:
1. Blend all the ingredients until smooth.
2. Serve.

Healthy Broccoli with Cheese Sauce

Ingredients:
- 6 cups broccoli florets
- 10 tbsp. milk
- 1.5 oz. Mexican cheese, crumbled
- 4 tsp. aji amarillo paste
- 6 pcs. saltine crackers
- cooking spray

Instructions:
1. Coat the broccoli florets lightly with cooking spray.
2. Place half of the florets in the air fryer basket and cook them for 8 minutes at 375°F.
3. Once cooked, repeat the process with the remaining florets.
4. In a blender, add milk, cheese, amarillo paste, along with saltines. Blend until the mixture becomes smooth.
5. Pour the sauce in a microwaveable bowl. Microwave the mixture for 30 seconds.
6. Serve the broccoli with the cheese sauce.

Broccoli Soup

Ingredients:
- 1 onion, chopped
- 1 lb. broccoli, chopped
- 1 small tomato, chopped
- 1 tbsp. grapeseed oil
- 1/2 cup unsweetened almond milk
- 16 oz. water
- 1/4 tsp. turmeric
- cayenne pepper, to taste

Instructions:
1. Put oil and onion in a medium pot. Saute over medium heat for about a couple of minutes.
2. Add the seasoning, tomato, and broccoli. Saute for 10 more minutes.
3. Add 6 ounces of water. Cover the pot and let it simmer for a couple more minutes.
4. Transfer the contents into a blender, followed by the remaining water and milk. Blend for a couple of minutes.
5. Pour back the blended ingredients into the pot.
6. Raise up the heat and boil for a couple of minutes.

Stir-Fried Cabbage and Apples

Ingredients:
- 1 shallot, thinly sliced
- 1/2 apple, cut into cubes
- 1/4 savoy cabbage, sliced thinly into strips
- 3–4 radishes, sliced thinly
- 1/2–1 tsp. coconut oil
- salt, to taste

Instructions:
1. Pour some coconut oil into a wok.
2. Add shallot and cook until translucent.
3. Add the cabbage, radish, and apples to the wok.
4. Stir-fry for about 5 minutes. Don't overcook.
5. Add salt to taste.
6. Serve while warm.

Broccoli-Kale with Avocado Toppings Rice Bowl

Ingredients:
- 1/2 avocado
- 2 cups kale
- 1 cup broccoli florets
- 1/2 cup cooked brown rice
- 1 tsp. plum vinegar
- 2 tsp. tamari
- sea salt, to taste

Instructions:
1. In a small pot, simmer broccoli florets, and kale in about 3 tbsp. of water. Cook for 2 minutes.
2. Add tamari, vinegar, and cooked brown rice. Stir to combine.
3. Transfer pot contents into a medium-sized bowl and top with sliced avocado; sprinkle a dash of sea salt to taste.
4. Serve immediately.

Vitamin D-Rich Recipes

Roasted Mushroom Soup

Ingredients:
- 1 lb. mushrooms, chopped
- 1 onion, chopped
- 3 garlic cloves, chopped
- 4 cups vegetable broth
- 2 cups milk
- 1 tbsp. olive oil
- salt
- pepper

Instructions:
1. Preheat the oven to 375°F.
2. Combine the olive oil, onion, garlic, and mushrooms in a baking dish. Season with pepper and salt.
3. Roast for 25 minutes.
4. In a pot, combine the roasted vegetables, vegetable broth, and milk. Bring to a boil then reduce to a simmer.
5. Use an immersion blender to blend the soup until smooth.
6. Serve with a dollop of milk and freshly ground pepper.

This recipe features mushrooms, which are a good source of vitamin D. The soup is also fortified with vitamin D-rich milk.

Avocado and Egg Salad

Ingredients:
- 6 hard boiled eggs
- 1 avocado
- 1/4 cup red onion, chopped
- 1/4 cup celery, chopped
- 1/4 cup mayonnaise
- 1 tbsp. white vinegar
- salt
- pepper

Instructions:
1. In a bowl, combine the eggs, avocado, red onion, celery, mayonnaise, and white vinegar. Season with salt and pepper.
2. Serve on whole wheat bread or crackers.

This recipe features eggs, which are a good source of vitamin D. The avocado provides healthy fats and fiber.

Spicy Tuna Salad

Ingredients:
- 1 can tuna
- 1 avocado
- 1 tomato
- 1/4 cup onion, diced
- 1 tbsp. olive oil
- 1 tbsp. lemon juice
- salt
- pepper

Instructions:
1. In a bowl, combine the tuna, avocado, tomato, onion, olive oil, and lemon juice. Season with salt and pepper.
2. Serve on whole wheat bread or crackers.

This recipe features tuna, which is a good source of vitamin D. The salad also includes avocado and tomato, both of which are good sources of healthy fats.

Salmon with Sweet Potato and Kale

Ingredients:
- 1 lb. salmon
- 1 head of kale
- 1 sweet potato
- 1 tbsp. olive oil
- salt
- pepper

Instructions:
1. Preheat the oven to 350°F.
2. Remove the stem from the kale and chop it into small pieces.
3. Peel the sweet potato and cut it into small cubes.
4. Combine the salmon, kale, sweet potato, and olive oil in a baking dish. Season with salt and pepper.
5. Bake for 20-25 minutes, or until the salmon is cooked through.

This recipe features salmon, which is a good source of vitamin D. The sweet potato provides beta-carotene while the kale provides calcium.

No-Fuss Tuna Casserole

Ingredients:
- 1-5 oz. can tuna, drained
- 1 can cream of chicken soup, condensed
- 3 cups macaroni, cooked
- 1-1/2 cups fried onions
- 1 cup Cheddar cheese, shredded

Instructions:
1. Preheat the oven to 350°F.
2. Prepare a 9x13-inch baking dish. Use that to mix the macaroni, tuna, and soup. Top it with cheese.
3. Bake for 25 minutes or until the casserole is bubbly.
4. Sprinkle it with fried onions. Put back in the oven and leave for 5 more minutes.
5. Serve and enjoy while hot.

Fried Eggs and Vegetables

Ingredients:
- coconut oil
- 1 pack frozen vegetable mix
- 3-4 pcs. eggs
- pepper
- salt
- a few stalks of spinach
- spice mix or preferred spices
- desired fruit

Instructions:
1. Heat up a frying pan and pour coconut oil.
2. Add the vegetables.
3. Add eggs, followed by salt, pepper, and spices, according to your taste preference.
4. Add spinach.
5. Stir fry until cooked. Don't overcook the vegetables.
6. Serve while warm.

Exotic Empanadas

Ingredients:
- 3 ox. lean ground beef
- 3 oz. mushrooms, chopped
- 1/4 cup onion, chopped finely
- 2 tsp. garlic, chopped finely
- 1/2 cup tomatoes, chopped
- 1/4 tsp. paprika
- 6 green olives, chopped
- 1/4 tsp. ground cumin
- 1/8 tsp. ground cinnamon
- 8 square gyoza wrappers
- 1 large egg, beaten
- 1 tbsp. olive oil

Instructions:
1. Take a skillet and add oil. Heat the oil over a medium-high flame.
2. Once heated, add ground beef and onion into it. Stir the mixture to crumble for 3 minutes.
3. Once the beef mixture starts turning brown, add chopped mushrooms and cook for 6 minutes. Stir occasionally.
4. Once the mushrooms turn brown, add other ingredients like olives, garlic, paprika, grounded cinnamon, and cumin.
5. Cook the mixture for 3 minutes or until the mushrooms become very tender. Add tomatoes and cook for another minute. Stir occasionally.
6. Once done, transfer the mixture to a bowl. Let it cool for 5 minutes.
7. On a flat surface arrange gyoza wrappers. Fill about 1-1/2 tablespoons of the filling in the center of the wrappers.
8. Brush the edges of each wrapper with a beaten egg. Fold

each of the gyoza wrappers and use your hand to seal the edges.

9. Take the air fryer basket and place four empanadas in a single layer.

10.   Cook them for 7 minutes at 400°F or until they turn brown. Repeat the procedure with the remaining empanadas.

11.   Serve and enjoy while hot.

Salmon with Avocados and Brussels Sprout

Ingredients:
- 2 lbs. of salmon filet, divided into 4 pieces
- 1 tsp. ground cumin
- 1 tsp. onion powder
- 1 tsp. paprika powder
- 1/2 tsp. garlic powder
- 1 tsp. chili powder
- Himalayan sea salt
- black pepper, freshly grounded

Avocado sauce:
- 2 chopped avocados
- 1 lime, squeezed for the juice
- 1 tbsp. extra-virgin olive oil
- 1 tbsp. fresh minced cilantro
- 1 diced small red onion
- 1 minced garlic clove
- Himalayan sea salt to taste
- black pepper, freshly grounded

Brussels sprout:
- 3 lbs. of Brussels sprout
- 1/2 cup raw honey
- 1/2 cup balsamic vinegar
- 1/2 cup melted coconut oil
- 1 cup dried cranberries
- Himalayan sea salt to taste
- black pepper, freshly grounded

Instructions:
To make the salmon and avocado sauce:
1. Combine cumin, onion, chili powder, garlic, and paprika seasoned with salt and pepper. Mix well before dry rubbing on the salmon.
2. Place the salmon in the fridge for 30 minutes.

3. Preheat the grill.
4. In a bowl, mash avocado until the texture becomes smooth. Pour in all the remaining ingredients and mix thoroughly.
5. Grill salmon for 5 minutes on each side or until cooked.
6. Drizzle avocado on cooked salmon.

To make the Brussel sprouts:
1. Preheat the oven to 375°F.
2. Mix Brussels sprouts with coconut oil. Season with salt and pepper.
3. Place vegetables on a baking sheet and roast for about 30 minutes.
4. In a separate pan, combine vinegar and honey.
5. Simmer in slow heat until it boils and thickens.
6. Drizzle them on top of the Brussels Sprouts.
7. Serve with the salmon.

Pomegranate Refreshing Smoothie

Ingredients:
- 2 grapefruits
- 1/2 pomegranate
- 3 large collard leaves
- 1 cup coconut water

Instructions:
1. Put all ingredients in a blender.
2. Blend well.
3. Serve and enjoy.

CONCLUSION

As you've learned, Osteopenia is a condition characterized by low bone density. While it is not as severe as osteoporosis, it can still lead to an increased risk of fractures.

You can do several things to help prevent or manage osteopenia, including getting enough calcium and vitamin D, exercising, and eating a healthy diet.

This 3-week guide provides tips on how to get started with making dietary changes to help manage osteopenia.

You'll learn about the importance of calcium and vitamin D, bone-healthy foods to eat, and ways to reduce your risk of falls. By following this guide, you'll be on your way to making lifestyle changes that may help you manage bone health.

While this guide provides some basic information on osteopenia, it is not intended to replace the advice of a healthcare professional. If you have any concerns about your bone health, talk to your doctor.

If you enjoyed this guide, please leave a review. Best wishes for managing your osteopenia.

Reference and Helpful Links

"Osteopenia (Low Bone Density): What Is It, Prevention, Symptoms, Causes & Treatment." Cleveland Clinic, https:// my.clevelandclinic.org/health/diseases/21855-osteopenia. Accessed 20 June 2022.

Varacallo, Matthew, et al. "Osteopenia." StatPearls, StatPearls Publishing, 2022. PubMed, http://www.ncbi.nlm.nih.gov/books/ NBK499878/. Accessed 20 June 2022.

"What Women Need to Know." Bone Health & Osteoporosis Foundation, https://www.bonehealthandosteoporosis.org/ preventing-fractures/general-facts/what-women-need-to-know/. Accessed 20 June 2022.

"You've Heard of Osteoporosis. What About Osteopenia?" Hospital for Special Surgery, https://www.hss.edu/article_what-is-osteopenia.asp. Accessed 20 June 2022.

Made in the USA
Monee, IL
17 March 2023

30010919R00026